Candida Cleanse Guide for Women

Beat Yeast and Candidiasis

By: Alma Williams

ISBN-13: 978-0692230251

PUBLISHERS NOTES

Disclaimer

This publication is intended to provide helpful and informative material. It is not intended to diagnose, treat, cure, or prevent any health problem or condition, nor is intended to replace the advice of a physician. No action should be taken solely on the contents of this book. Always consult your physician or qualified health-care professional on any matters regarding your health and before adopting any suggestions in this book or drawing inferences from it.

The author and publisher specifically disclaim all responsibility for any liability, loss or risk, personal or otherwise, which is incurred as a consequence, directly or indirectly, from the use or application of any contents of this book.

Any and all product names referenced within this book are the trademarks of their respective owners. None of these owners have sponsored, authorized, endorsed, or approved this book.

Always read all information provided by the manufacturers' product labels before using their products. The author and publisher are not responsible for claims made by manufacturers.

Paperback Edition

Manufactured in the United States of America

DEDICATION

To all the women that want to stop buying those creams and antibiotic pills in the pharmacy and want to find a natural way to deal with their yeast infections. This is the answer for you!

"Young women, adolescent girls, are more subject to infection, sometimes at a rate of six times that of boys. That tells you a lot about the vulnerability of women."

Stephen Lewis

TABLE OF CONTENTS

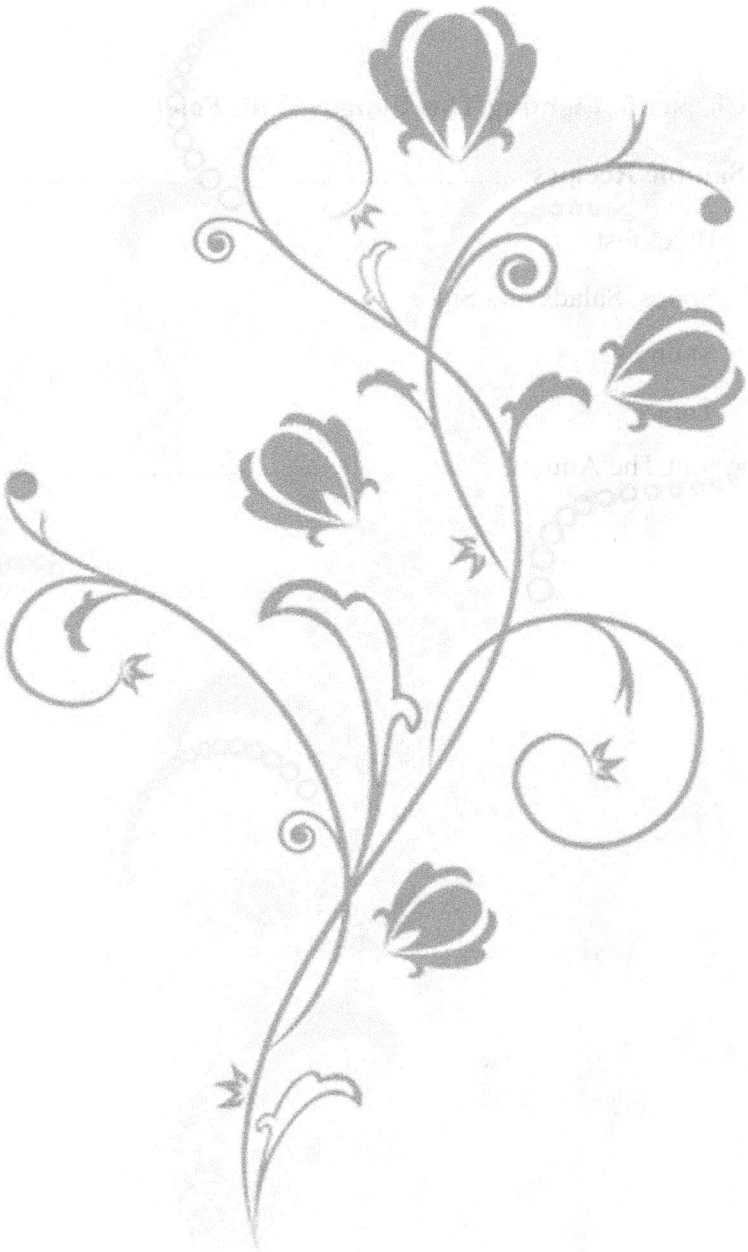

CHAPTER 1

WHAT YOU NEED TO KNOW ABOUT CANDIDA

Candida Albicans affects different parts of the body; the disease usually develops in the mouth, genitals, skin, nails and the digestive tract. When the fungus grows in the mouth, it is called thrush – *this is mostly found in infants*.

You can recognize it by the bluish-red patches that would be visible all over the tongue. This infection sometimes travels down the throat inflaming the digestive tract as well.

When it breeds in the vagina, it causes *vaginitis moniliasis*, which is commonly known as a yeast infection. This causes inflammation of the vulva and the walls of the vagina with itching and burning sensations.

When the infection affects the penis, it is normally characterized by the inflammation of the head of the penis. It has been observed that circumcised men are less likely to catch the infection than those who are not circumcised. Genital infection is often transmitted through sexual intercourse.

On the skin, it is recognizable as a angry-red rash which is often scaly similar to diaper rash. On finger and toenails it appears as a painful and red swelling that unless treated it could form pus.

Infants are often infected with this fungus in the diaper area; this is characterized by angry red painful swelling in the groin area.

As mentioned earlier, it can enter the blood stream and attack internal organs:

Where it attacks the kidneys, the main symptom would be pain and presence of blood in the urine.

Where it affects the eyes, the person develops blurred vision and acute pain.

When the heart is the affected organ, it develops heart murmurs and/or valve damage.

When it affects the lungs, Candida Albicans is characterized by bloody sputum

When it affects the brain, the symptoms can be very severe such as seizures and sudden changes in behavior and mental activity.

TREATMENT IS WITHIN REACH

The good news is that the Candida Albicans can be treated with OTC drugs, or natural approaches. In most cases, anti-fungal ointment and drugs can immediately check and reverse the condition.

More serious infections, especially those that affect internal organs, might require IV medication. Overall, keeping the skin clean and dry can deter the fungus from breeding and prevent infection recurrence.

HAVE NO FEAR

Candida is a fungus that lives in every one.

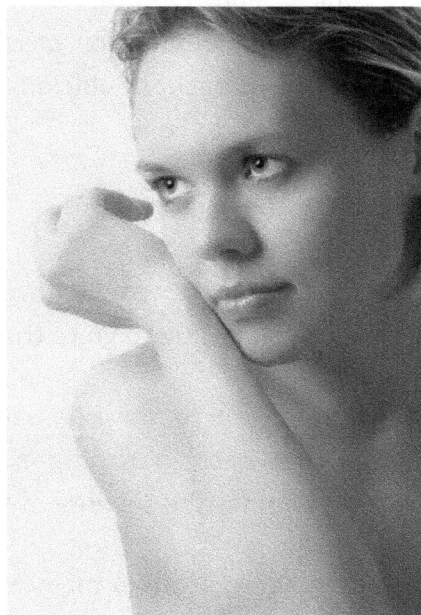

Normally it is harmless and we have no problems with it. However, when the digestive system goes even a little off then this is when this fungus goes to town, literally.

In many cases, just taking care of your digestion could get you rid of your Candida symptoms.

In other cases when excessive use of antibiotics could have triggered the out-of-control multiplying of the fungus, the use of probiotics would be exceptionally useful. Side-by-side with introducing digestion-enhancing enzymes and probiotics, you should always aim at boosting your immune system.

When the fungal infection is persistent, you could move to medication both topical and internal and eliminate any inhibiting fungal growth and colonization or look at some of the more natural approaches including my top recommendations in chapters to come.

TESTING FOR CANDIDIASIS

If you think you or your partner could have a candidiasis infection, it may be that you decide to go to the doctor.

Your natural inclination may be to move on and start treating without examination, however, obtaining a final exam is worth it, because it determines the severity of the infection.

If you go to the doctor, there are two main ways to test for candidiasis infection. The first is by a microscopic examination. This analysis is done using a photo-microscope and a sample.

A sample is obtained by scraping with a cotton swab the affected area. The sample is placed on a bar and a drop of potassium hydroxide solution 10% (KOH) is added. This solution dissolves the skin cells but leaves the candidiasis cells intact. The doctor can then watch these candida cells through the microscope, if they exist.

The second method of testing for candida is culture. It is carried out by rubbing cotton on the affected area and then streaking the specimen on a culture medium.

This culture is then placed in a chamber or culture and incubated for several days at a temperature of 36.9 ° C (98.6 ° F). In the culture of candidiasis , the colony of bacteria is growing rapidly because it is the perfect environment.

The visual characteristics of what develops, such as color, give an idea of what develops. A look at the sample through a microscope can be done or a study by a more sophisticated analysis method to obtain a result.

Your doctor may request a blood test for uric acid levels that may indicate the presence of a candidiasis infection.

A full analysis will show digestive flora in your body and seeks digestive disorders that may be related to candidiasis.

Your doctor may advise you to have laboratory tests that make diagnostics for Candida antigens in your blood. This tests for antibody levels of candida in the body.

It is a way to determine how you are susceptible to the candidiasis infection.

SPOTTING SYMPTOMS

Did you know that the Candida fungal infection can release about 70 different types of toxins in your body? This is why Candida symptoms are many and often seemingly unrelated:

Bloating, flatulence and acute abdominal pains

Fatigue – you only want to sleep, or lie down

Headaches that develop suddenly without any obvious trigger

Anxiety – many people develop symptoms of anxiety

Mood swings

Rectal itching and localized burning sensation

Sudden uncontrollable **craving for sweets**

Diarrhea

Acne – you could develop a sudden burst of acne

Inflammation of the sinus – which also aggravates your headaches and leads to migraines

Vaginitis – when yeast infection attacks the genitals of a female

Depression – there is often inexplicable mood swings coupled with depression and anxiety attacks. *We elaborate more on this in later chapters.*

Poor memory – the memory and clarity of thought is influenced when the fungus spreads to the brain through blood

Sensitivity to smell – you will find that suddenly you do not tolerate strong smells – good or bad.

Sore throat – this is a sore throat that does not go away, especially with antibiotic treatment. This is the extension of thrush, when left untreated for a long time as the fungus spreads down the digestive tract.

Craving for alcohol – it is often seen that one of the most dangerous Candida symptoms is attraction to alcohol, which in many cases leads to alcoholism.

Indigestion – this in turn gives rise to flatulence, bloating feelings that we spoke about a little earlier.

Learning difficulties – it is well known that learning difficulties is among the regular Candida symptoms.

Muscle weakness – you will often experience a total weakness; as if someone drained out all your energy and you need to make an effort even to raise your hand.

Acid reflux – this is once again tied to poor digestion, which is one of the leading Candida symptoms

Candida can attack your digestive system, nervous system, cardio-vascular system, musculoskeletal system, urinary tract, reproductive system, lymphatic system, respiratory system and endocrine system among others.

The symptoms you may experience could vary according to the part of the body worst affected.

CHAPTER 2

START TREATING YOUR INFECTION

Why take an antibiotic if you do not need it

With a strong immune system, you can fight infections in about ten days. With an antibiotic, you can fight infections in about ten days. If this has peaked your interest, you will love the natural treatment methods and immunity boosters that I am going to share with you.

SIDE NOTE ON ANTIBIOTICS:

Unless your doctor has examined you for a bacterial infection, an antibiotic is not appropriate. If you prescribed, it is important to

Take the prescription to the end and not to stop. The premature termination will only bad bacteria stronger and they defeat the good bacteria.

This will allow bacterial infections candida to thrive in your vagina. You could develop a resistant infection that will be more difficult to treat, make you very sick, and that could be a nightmare to remove.

Without proper examination of tissue culture, it is possible that we will be prescribed an antibiotic for a fungal infection.

And, believe it or not, it happens often. In this case, the antibiotic does not help. Your condition will worsen, and it is possible that the doctor may prescribe a stronger antibiotic. They just make the fungal infection worse.

By the time the test results arrive, you might be really sick, and it could take weeks to months to process. Everything is preventable by getting the correct initial diagnosis.

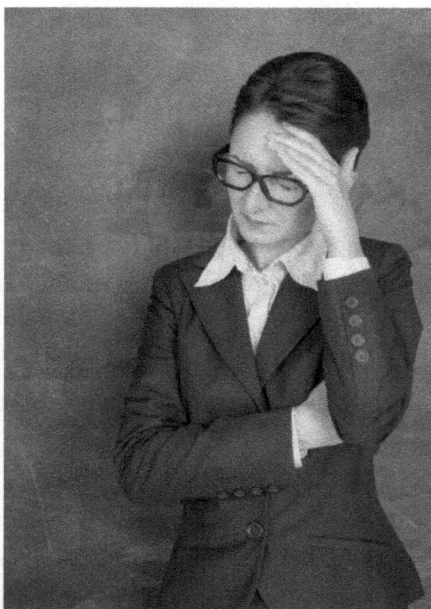

Now I know it is not at the forefront of your mind, but you should not to use antibacterial soap to wash your vagina. The excessive use of antibacterial soaps cause an antibiotic-induced candidiasis infection.

More problematic is the potential that the abuse of antibacterial products may reduce the effectiveness of your natural immune system, or probably stop working correctly. This can become a weakened immune system.

NATURAL TREATMENT METHODS:

There are numerous natural remedies to choose from the all-natural list of Candida treatments. The good news is that almost all can be found in your kitchen pantry.

Apple cider vinegar – this is one of the best natural ingredients you could utilize as Candida treatments. You could use it liberally as food and as a topical douche. This is an extremely potent cure for vaginal Candida yeast infection as well as other fungal infections such as dandruff, and skin infections.

Oregano – a favorite spice for many, the oil of oregano (available as essential oil) can be used in minimal quantity in salad dressings or sauces. Many find it a little too strong; in such a case, you could add a few drops in a glass of water and take it as a medicine. Follow it with another glass of water to get you rid of the strong taste. This is among the best natural Candida treatments for thrush (mouth Candida infection), finger and toenails infection and skin infection. You can also apply the essential oil topically for better results.

Garlic – this is another highly potent anti-fungal natural food. It contains a number of sulphur compounds such as allicin, sally cysteine, and alliin among others, which makes it an extremely powerful anti-fungal agent. The best use is to add it crushed to your food wherever you find the occasion.

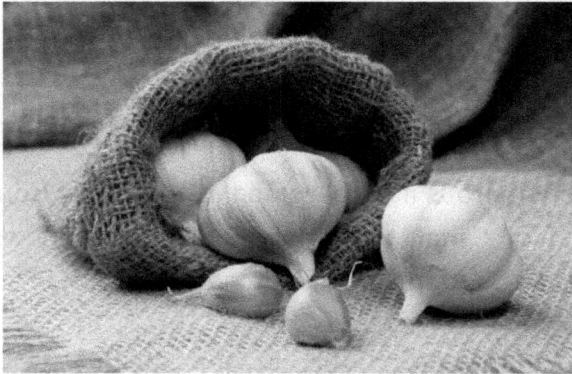

Cloves – tea made with cloves is an excellent natural anti-fungal treatment. This is a compound that works best when taken internally or applied externally. If you do not enjoy the pungent taste in your tea, try one drop diluted in a glass of water taken as medicine. You could also apply it directly especially to toe and finger nail and skin Candida infections.

Coconut oil – coconut oil contains caprylic acid, which has proved to be an excellent Candida treatment as it inhibits fungal growth both externally and internally. The best would be to use it raw in the form of high-quality virgin coconut oil.

If you do not like the specific flavor, you could settle for the deodorized (refined) version, which is best used in cooking. Ensure however, that you never buy hydrogenated oil as this is harmful to your health.

As you can see, there are plenty of all-natural Candida

treatments that you could use without much effort. Just introduce these foods into your daily diet and continue enjoying them even after you get rid of your fungal infections.

Side-by-side you need to consider supplementing your diet with probiotics and foods that enhance your immune system.

Probiotics promote the growth of the friendly bacteria in your body, which would in turn deter the overgrowth of Candida Albicans; while an enhanced immune system would stop it from spreading and colonizing.

WHY TRY THE CANDIDA DIET

The goal of being on the candida diet is to create an environment that does not support the overgrowth of candida and yeast. Candida occurs naturally in the digestive tract and we are not out to kill off all the candida in our bodies.

What we are concerned with is balancing the amount of candida occurring. When there is an overgrowth of candida, many of the body systems including the digestive system and immune system become weak. These systems must be re-strengthened in order to stop the overgrowth and re-balance the candida and yeast in our bodies.

If you have had an overgrowth of candida for a long time you have probably noticed many of these symptoms and others that the diet can help to solve very quickly:

constipation or diarrhea

chronic heartburn

chronic fatigue

bladder infections

migraines

depression and/or mood swings

food intolerances or sensitivities

leaky gut syndrome or irritable bowel syndrome symptoms

How Long Do I Stay on the Candida Diet?

This is a question many people want to know when they first find out they have an overgrowth of candida and start looking at the candida diet. I wish I could tell you an exact length of time or that there was an easy answer, but there isn't.

It depends on the severity of your condition and many other individual factors. It is possible for you to get relief of symptoms within two to four weeks of being on the candida diet or it may take several months. To completely regain your health can take even longer, possibly a year or more depending on the severity.

The good news is that being on the candida diet is an overall healthier way to eat and just because you get relief from symptoms doesn't mean you should go back to eating all the sugar, carbs and processed foods you want. You may get to a point where you can relax some of the restrictions, but you may decide that you feel so good eating healthier that you will continue to eat this way.

Determiners for you individually will be to look at what led to your overgrowth in the first place and how severe your condition has become. If you have made changes to your

lifestyle to reduce stress, stay away from antibiotics, cut out alcohol and excessive sugars from your diet, you may get to a point, after being on the diet for a period of time, where your candida is balanced.

You may then decide that while you should still avoid excessive sugar and refined foods, you may no longer need to adhere strictly to the candida diet.

Another determiner may be if you get relief from your symptoms, relax the candida diet and then see symptoms reappear. That will let you know that you need to continue on the diet longer. You may think you have killed off the excess candida in your body only to find it returns fairly quickly.

This can be due to the yeast being able grow roots into the blood vessels of the intestines which makes it harder to kill off and allow it to get enough sugar to keep it alive.

Success on the candida diet can also vary according to if you cleansed your system before starting the diet or not. This can be achieved by fasting, using an enema, eating detoxing herbs and drinking lots of non-chlorinated water and vegetable juices. The chapter on Candida Cleanse will give you many additional cleansing suggestions.

REPLACING YOUR FRIENDLY BACTERIA

Another consideration in determining how long to stay on the candida diet is the importance of repopulating your friendly bacteria which in turns supports the health of the digestive system and immune system.

Candida and yeast kill off friendly bacteria in the intestine that are necessary for good digestive health. Probiotics such as acidophilus and bifidus can help support the intestinal tract by helping to create an environment for beneficial flora to thrive and prevent unfriendly microorganisms such as candida and yeast from growing.

If you are considering starting the Candida diet, my best advice to you is to not worry about how long you will have to be on it. I can attest to the relief a candida sufferer can achieve from being on the diet and taking probiotics and enzymes.

That kind of relief is worth any investment in time that you end up spending making diet and lifestyle changes. You will end up being a happier and healthier person.

Alma Williams

Eat This Not That on the Candida Cleanse Diet

The main culprit that has to be cut out of the diet is sugar since yeast feeds off sugar which allows it to multiply rapidly. Cutting sugar out of the diet helps to starve the candida and reduce its growth. This includes any type of refined brown sugar, molasses, white sugars, honey, and agave and foods that are broken down into sugars such as simple carbohydrates like potatoes, milk, fructose, white flour and alcohol.

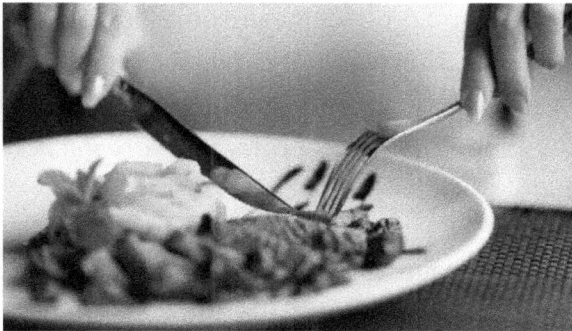

That would mean fruit, breads, condiments, sauces, and most processed foods are out. Caffeine should also be removed from the diet as there is some evidence that suggests it suppresses the immune system which needs to be in good shape to fight off candida.

Colon Cleanse

There are many types of cleanses for various organs such as liver, gallbladder and kidney and different sources recommend different ways to do these. One type of cleanse recommended for dealing with symptoms of candida is a colon cleanse. If you are in a position to do this type of cleanse, it can help get you started towards the candida diet by flushing out your colon which is where most of the internal candida grows. If you are in a situation such as holding a full time job that you can't take time off from, then this step may not be doable for you. A colon cleanse typically takes 3 days to a week to do.

Diet Cleanse

The alternative would be to make some drastic diet changes for 1 to 2 weeks. This would include cutting all sugar, white flour, cheese and yeast and anything else from your diet except raw and steamed, preferably organic, vegetables along with doing a liver flush.

For the cleanse stage of the candida diet, eating only non starchy vegetables will help starve the candida by denying it the sugar and mold it feeds on. It will also help absorb fungal toxins and flush them out of your body. Starchy vegetables such as potatoes, corn, sweet potatoes, yams and winter squash are not allowed in the candida diet and certainly not during the cleansing stage.

And of course be sure to drink lots of water during the cleansing stage. Doing the diet cleanse as the first step can help take drastic action towards reducing the overgrowth of candida and reducing the symptoms of candida.

Some people notice an increase of symptoms when first beginning the cleanse before they see improvement. As the yeast dies off it releases toxins that can create symptoms such as acne, headaches, fatigue, muscle or joint pain and swollen glands.

Don't let this get you down, remember it's always darkest before the dawn. Persevere through the entire cleansing process and it will pay off in the end.

The cleansing stage of the candida diet is more restrictive than the regular diet. After doing the cleanse for 1-2 weeks, you can take the next step by going to the candida diet which allows you to add foods such as whole grains, quinoa, brown rice, avocados, lean meats, eggs and nuts. Stevia, which is a plant-based sweetener, is also allowable on the candida diet.

Liver Flush

There are a variety of types of liver flushes, but basically they clean toxins out of the liver and gallbladder and contain ingredients such as water, garlic, ginger, olive oil, Epsom salts, a variety of juices, herbs, and enzymes. The type of liver flush you choose to use may depend on other conditions that you have, so check with your health care practitioner to make sure what you use is safe for you.

Other Natural Solutions for the Cleanse

Along with the vegetable diet and liver cleanse, you can build up your digestive system and immune system by taking high quality probiotics. The candida and yeast kill off friendly bacteria in the intestine that are necessary for good digestive health. Probiotics such as acidophilus and bifidus can help support the intestinal tract by helping to create an environment for beneficial flora to thrive and prevent unfriendly microorganisms such as candida and yeast from growing.

There are other natural solutions that can be helpful during the cleansing stage. Natural anti-fungals can be used. This could include oregano oil or garlic. Anti-microbials such as wormwood or thujone have been used successfully during the fungal stage of candida as well as pau d'arco.

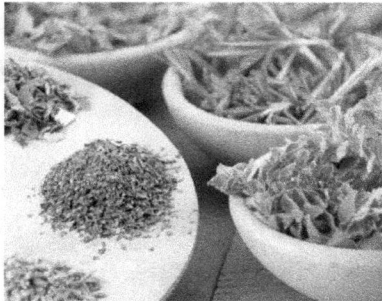

Each person's body responds differently, so get good at checking in with your body to see how you feel. Some people after the cleanse will be able to reintroduce some foods that are not allowed during the cleanse back into their diets and won't be able to tolerate other foods.

One approach is to introduce one type of food back into the diet at a time after cleansing and listen to your body to see if you feel better or worse.

CHAPTER 3

BREAKING THE SIDE EFFECTS OF CANDIDA

The fungus is able to penetrate the membrane lining of the digestive tract, break through the intestinal wall and enter the bloodstream. This systemic candida infection can then travel to other parts of the body and secrete over 70 harmful toxins into the bloodstream. The liver is supposed to detoxify blood, but if candida invades the liver, it is not able to do an optimal job.

When the blood that feeds the brain is affected, brain functioning can be affected.

One of the symptoms of candida affecting the bloodstream feeding the brain is depression. Other neurological functions that can be affected include memory, anxiety, mood swings and reasoning ability.

Another possible reason that Candida could be a cause of depression is that the overgrowth reduces the body's capability of absorbing magnesium and magnesium deficiency has been linked to being a cause of depression.

The candida diet can be an effective way of dealing with not only the physical symptoms of candida, but also depression and other mood and emotional symptoms.

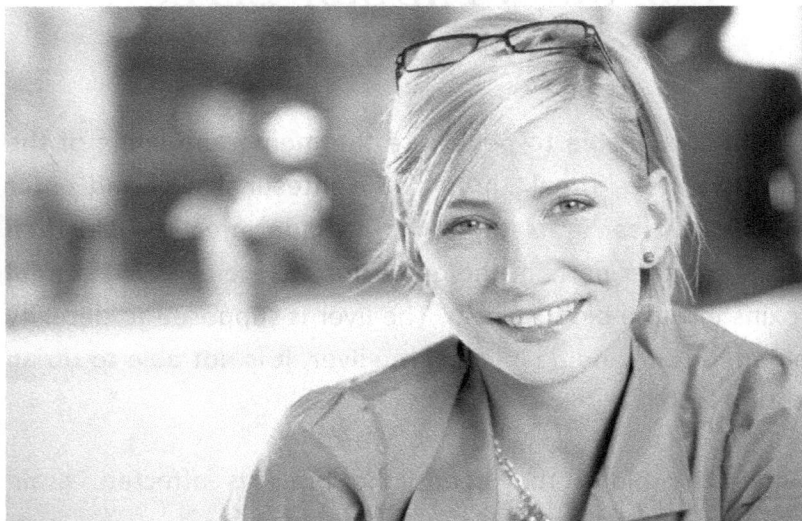

Symptoms that appear as depressive symptoms may be apparent in candida sufferers because of attitude. If you see all the foods you can't eat, are suffering with physical discomforts and pain that you don't think will go away, and feel your lifestyle is limited by having to be on the Candida diet, this can lead to negativity, irritability, mood swings and other signs that look like depression. If the depression is a result of the physical changes in the body, the candida diet can be helpful.

According to the Mayo Clinic, eating a healthy diet high in vegetables and fruits, whole grains and healthy fats has been shown to reduce the risks of depression symptoms. Also negative moods can be associated with low blood sugar which eating healthy foods at regular intervals can assist in keeping balanced.

Getting enough omega-3 fatty acids in the diet from foods such as tuna, lake trout, blue green algae, olive oil, wild rice, spinach, chia seeds, salmon, herring, flaxseed, walnuts, edamame, soybean oil and kale, can improve brain health and help with depression.

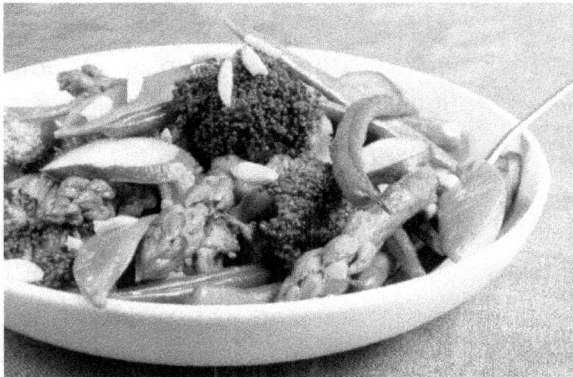

Taking probiotics such as acidophilus and bifidus and taking digestive enzymes can also help address the overgrowth of candida in the body and aid in digestion to get the most benefit of the foods you eat. Addressing the overgrowth through diet, supplements and an anti-fungal can help with reducing the problem which in turn reduces the symptoms of candida.

Depressive symptoms coming from either a physical cause or more from a negative attitude and being "down" about a drastic change in lifestyle that are not responding to the diet alone need to be addressed by other means. Emotional outlook and attitude as well as stress can have an enormous affect on everything else you do and on your health. Without addressing the emotional side, it's like only seeing half the picture. Here are some examples of things to consider.

Get Positive and Proactive

Most people living with Candida have run into a negative experience in the medical community that has contributed to their frustration and negative attitude. A great many doctors in conventional medicine do not recognize systemic candida as a physical problem and dismiss the symptoms as being caused by a candida overgrowth.

If you have had an experience like this, remember you are not alone and keep looking for a health care provider who does not discount your symptoms and will work with you to help overcome them. This may mean searching outside the conventional medical community and finding a holistic or naturopathic doctor.

Positive thinking has an effect on brain health and can help with reducing stress. Thinking positive thoughts about yourself and your situation helps build self confidence which can have an effect on your performance and outlook on life.

Finding a way to stay positive so that you can advocate for yourself is important. Whether it is using affirmations, meditation, yoga or some other type of exercise or finding a support group, find something that can help keep your spirits from sagging.

EFT

EFT, Emotional Freedom Technique, has proved useful for some people in dealing with negative emotions, food cravings and keeping a positive attitude.

EFT works on the same energy meridians as acupuncture, but without the needles. It involves tapping your fingers on certain points of the body in association with a particular problem, negative emotion or event. This technique is said to clear the emotional block in the body's energetic system so that mind and body are back in balance. The techniques used are outside the scope of this book, but you can find many good resources online, at your bookstore or at your library.

Supplementation

Curcumin, found in turmeric, has been the basis of much research and found to have benefit for enhancing memory, as an anti-inflammatory, for enhancing nerve growth in areas of the brain and as an antidepressant. It is also being studied and used in relation to treating Alzheimer's. Adding turmeric to dishes may help some people ward off depressive symptoms.

St. John's Wart is another natural substance that has been found useful by many people for mild to moderate depressive symptoms.

S-Adenosyl Methionine or SAM-e, is found naturally in the body and is thought to increase serotonin and dopamine levels making SAM-e supplements helpful to some for depression.

Of course, you should always check with your health care provider before taking these kinds of supplements especially if you are on medications to make sure they are safe for you to take.

If you suspect your Candida is your cause of depression, I urge you to try some or all of the solutions above. Depression can be very debilitating and is counteractive to improving your health. If you already are dealing with the symptoms of Candida, then life is hard enough for you right now without adding depression to it. Know that there is help available and you are not alone in searching for a way to deal with your symptoms of Candida.

CHAPTER 4

GETTING RID OF CANDIDA

Yeast infections do not discriminate. Anyone, men, women, children, and babies, can get one. Newborn infants might be infected during delivery.

Diabetics are more prone, as the sugar in their urine provides a good medium for the growth of yeast. (Anyone who bakes bread knows this.) Yeast exists everywhere, including our bodies. The organism resides naturally in miniscule amounts in the intestines.

When a fungus known as Candida grows to abnormally high levels, a yeast infection develops. Illness, antibiotic use, and other conditions can result in the proliferation of the fungus. The first signs are mild, and the afflicted person feels no pain. However, yeast grows at a rapid rate.

Once symptoms develop, it is vital to get medical attention. It's important to know about the various types of yeast infections and their symptoms.

Once you have gained better knowledge about the various types of infections, their root causes and their symptoms, you are well on your way to be better able to eliminate your excess Candida levels entirely.

INFECTION TYPES AND CAUSES

Vaginal Yeast Infection

It's estimated that 75% of women have at least one vaginal yeast infection. This disorder is officially known as vulvovaginal candidiasis because both the vagina and the surrounding vulva are affected.

The most frequently-observed sign is brutal itching. Burning, tenderness, swelling, inflamed tissues, a clear to white discharge which may appear lumpy, uncomfortable urination, and pain during intercourse are all symptoms of a vaginal yeast infection.

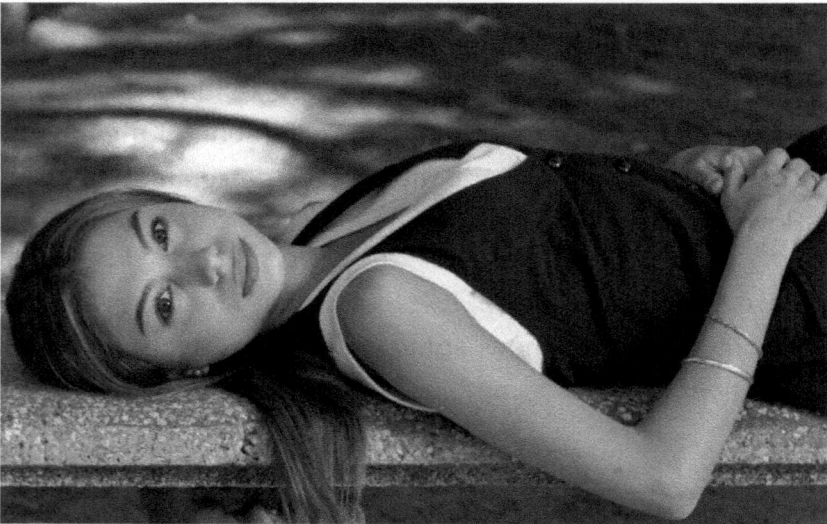

Since 12% to 15% of men may contract the infection following unprotected intercourse with a woman suffering from the disorder, it's important to begin treatment.

The causes are varied: the physical changes that accompany pregnancy, diabetes, immune system deficiency, birth control pills, menstruation, unprotected sex, and changes in hormone levels. Expectant mothers can rest assured that a vaginal yeast infection won't affect the pregnancy, but the unpleasant symptoms make treatment desirable.

Skin and Nail Yeast Infection

Candida Albicans is the infection-causing culprit here. This variety can manifest itself anywhere. Since yeast likes moist areas, sufferers may have an itchy red rash under their arms, between fingers and toes, in the lower abdomen and groin, under the breasts, and anywhere else where folds retain moisture.

Breast-feeding mothers can "catch" the infection from an infant with an oral yeast infection (see below). Breast infections can be quite painful and may be accompanied by burning, blisters, and itching.

Affected nails change in color to yellow or white, thicken, become crumbly and split, and may detach from the nail bed.

Cuts and sores may result in a skin infection. People most at risk are obese (there is more skin surface to be affected), have diabetes, are over 60, have a deficient immune system, wear shoes that make feet moist or sweaty, have hangnails or ingrown toenails, and reside or work where it is hot and humid.

Treatment is important, as the infection can spread. If left untreated, nail infections can permanently damage the nail or nail bed.

Thrush

Thrush, or oral yeast infection, is caused by Monilia Albicans and Candida. As it proliferates in the mouth and throat, white patches form on the tongue, on the roof of the mouth, inside the cheeks, and on the gums and lips.

Bleeding can occur if the patches are wiped away or damaged during the course of tooth brushing or eating. An uncomfortable ulcer may be visible. Cracks on the corners of the mouth, which are quite sore, can occur.

It is possible for the infection to spread to the throat and esophagus (esophagitis), making eating and drinking painful and difficult. Other symptoms include loss of taste and crankiness in babies.

Women who take birth control pills, which result in inadequate resistance to Candida, are at risk for developing thrush.

Another cause is antibiotic use. This type of medication eradicates not only disease-causing bacteria but the healthy variety that we need for proper digestion and the prevention of an explosion of yeast in our bodies.

Systemic Yeast Infection

If the fungus makes its way into the bloodstream, digestive system, or respiratory tract, a systemic yeast infection is the result. This serious disorder is characterized by muscle pain,

tiredness, changes in bowel movements, breathing difficulties, and dizziness. People whose immune systems do not function properly due to other medical conditions have a greater tendency to acquire a systemic yeast infection. Treatment is vital, for serious consequences can develop, and the condition might prove fatal if left untreated.

There are at least as many treatments for yeast infections as there are types of the malady. Oral and topical medications are widely used. Many effectively treat the condition, but some (especially in the case of nail infections) take a long time to show improvement.

Azoles are used for the treatment of systemic yeast infection, and a number of antifungal creams and locations provide relief for vaginal, skin, and nail types. Oral antifungal medications in the form of lozenges, tablets, or liquids are standard thrush remedies.

Now that you are familiar with the various types of yeast infections and the effects they have on people of all ages, you're in a position to make an intelligent treatment choice.

Treating Candida Infections Naturally

Don't forget many things can cause Candida yeast infections, including certain antibiotics (which kill the friendly bacteria that keep Candida in check), the use of oral contraceptives, steroidal medications and excess consumption of sugar. In addition, certain health conditions, such as a weakened immune system, diabetes or liver problems, can predispose people to the overgrowth of Candida yeast.

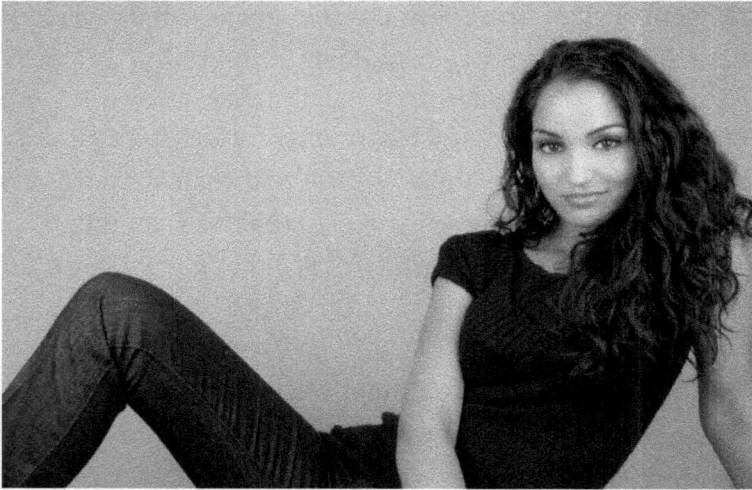

There are important questions to ask yourself if you suspect a Candida infection. Those questions include:

Have I taken a broad spectrum antibiotic for at least two months out of the year? Broad spectrum antibiotics include such commonly prescribed medications as Keflex, ampicillin, amoxicillin and Bactrim.

Have I used tetracycline or other antibiotics to treat acne for a month or more?

Have I taken birth control pills for more than two years?

Have I taken prednisone or other cortisone drugs for more than two weeks?

Do I notice my symptoms worsening when the weather is damp, muggy or humid?

Are my symptoms worse when I am around perfume, smoke, paint fumes or chemicals?

Natural treatments for Candida yeast infections can be very effective. When using supplements to treat a candid infection it is best to start with small doses and gradually increase those doses. That is because as Candida are killed, they can release toxins that can trigger an autoimmune response. This can result in a temporary worsening of symptoms. Most people begin to notice an improvement or lessening of symptoms within two to four weeks of starting treatment.

The Role of Diet

Diet is thought to play an important role in preventing and treating Candida infections. When adjusting your diet, be sure to eat plenty of healthy foods like beef, chicken, eggs, fish, yogurt, vegetables, nuts and seeds.

Foods to be avoided include refined and simple sugars. It is best to avoid sugars of all kinds, including white and brown sugars, honey, molasses and grain based sweeteners. It is also a good idea to eat plenty of raw garlic, and add it to foods for extra flavor.

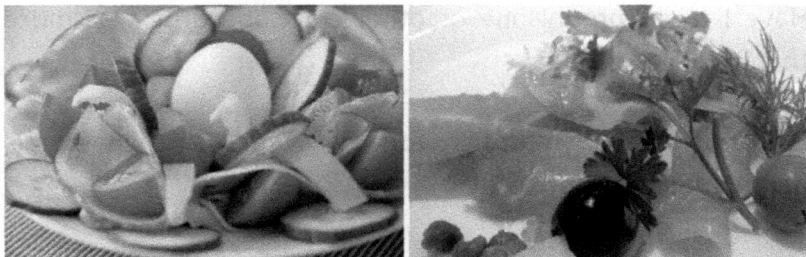

Milk and dairy products should be avoided, as should fruit, mushrooms and alcohol. It is important to avoid foods that contain yeast, including breads, cakes, muffins and baked goods.

Nutritional Supplements and Vitamins

Supplementation with acidophilus probiotic is often recommended for a Candida infection. Acidophilus is effective at controlling Candida because it acidifies the intestinal tract and makes it less attractive to the Candida organism.

Enteric-coated volatile oils have also been shown to be effective natural ways to treat a Candida yeast infection. Capsules containing oregano oil, peppermint oil and other volatile oils can help prevent and treat the overgrowth of Candida. Treatment with volatile oils should continue for a minimum of several months, and the standard dosage is two capsules twice a day. It is important not to take the oils directly, only in capsule forms, since the pure volatile oils can be toxic.

Enteric-coated garlic capsules can also be effective against Candida. Garlic is best used in combination with other encapsulated essential oils. Taking one capsule twice a day along with the essential oil capsules is the best approach.

*The best Diet is
the one you will
actually follow...*

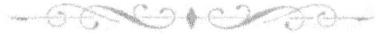

CHAPTER 5

FIGHTING THIS FUNGUS WITH FOOD

Balancing candida does not mean going hungry, just rethinking how we eat. A candida diet may seem restrictive to some at first, but with some research and creativity you can make delicious meals that fit within the diet's parameters.

You may find it helpful to take some digestive enzymes and probiotics with cooked food as well for better digestion. Promoting and providing good flora in the digestive tract is a must for keeping the candida balanced. Getting nutrition from food is only as good as one can digest.

My aim is to keep carbohydrates and sugar low while finding meals that are satisfying. The idea is to feed ourselves and not the candida. I like to think of candida as an unwanted house guest; I won't kick it out, but I don't need to feed it its favorite food either! A candida diet helps achieve this goal and finding new recipes that fit with the diet is a great place to start.

One of the main things to remember when on the candida diet is to eat fresh food. Don't leave leftovers sitting in the fridge too long because the more it breaks down the more it becomes food for the candida. What we want is to deprive the candida of its food so it goes away. Freezing food for later use is fine.

Patience is really the key: While you can expect to see progress on your Candida Diet, the process getting your body back in balance is one that is very slow and time-consuming. Your body will be making adjustments and you will be making adjustments to your eating habits too.

So, do not expect miracles to take place overnight. Have patience and stick to the diet and you will see the results in due time and you will be much healthier and happier.

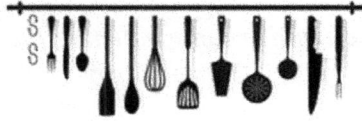

RECIPES

AVOCADO MORNING SMOOTHIE

"A deliciously green and creamy morning pick me up."

Servings: 1

Ingredients:

1/2 avocado

1 1/2 cups almond milk

2 tsp cinnamon

1/2 tsp pure vanilla extract

Liquid Stevia, to taste

1 cup ice

Directions:

1. Combine all ingredients into blender. Blend until smooth. Serve immediately.

COCONUT GRANOLA PARFAIT

"The crunchiness of granola paired with coconut and layered with Greek yogurt is a delectable morning treat."

Servings: 1

Ingredients:

1 cup oat bran

1 cup buckwheat

1/2 cup chia seeds

1/4 cup coconut oil

2 tsp. stevia (optional)

2 tbsp. cardamom

1/2 cup packed unsweetened shredded coconut

1 cup Greek yogurt

Directions:

1. Preheat the oven to 300 degrees F.

2. In a large bowl combine oat bran, buckwheat, chia seeds, coconut oil, stevia, if using and cardamom. Mix well.

3. Spread evenly on a baking sheet. Bake for 12 minutes, or until lightly brown and crunchy. Remove from oven.

4. Sprinkle the coconut evenly on top of the mixture and stir to combine. Put mixture back into oven and bake for an additional 12 minutes, until toasted. Remove from oven and cool.

5. In a large glass, layer the granola mixture with the Greek yogurt in 3 layers or as desired.

VEGETARIAN OMELET

"Eggs are an excellent way to start your day with a protein boost. The vegetable combination give this omelet great flavor and texture."

Servings: 1

Ingredients:

2 tbsp coconut oil

2 large eggs

2/3 cup chopped onion

2/3 cup chopped red pepper

1 cup chopped baby spinach

Directions:

1. In a small bowl, whisk eggs and set aside.

2. Add coconut oil to skillet and preheat over medium heat.

3. Add onions and peppers to skillet. Cook until soft and translucent. Add spinach and cook until soft.

4. Add eggs and cook for 3 to 4 minutes, or until eggs are done to your liking.

5. Remove from heat and serve immediately.

BUTTERNUT SQUASH SOUP

"The crunchiness of granola paired with coconut and layered with Greek yogurt is a delectable morning treat."

Servings: 1

Ingredients:

1 butternut squash, cubed (about 3 cups)

2 tsp olive oil

1 medium onion, sliced

1/2 teaspoon dried ginger

1/2 cup plain yogurt

Sea salt (optional)

Fresh parsley (optional)

Directions:

1. Cook cubes of squash in boiling water for about 10 minutes, or until soft.

2. Add olive oil to skillet and preheat over medium heat. Sauté onion until soft.

3. Add onions and squash to blender. Add water to blender as needed to blend until smooth and desired consistency.

4. Add blended squash mixture and ginger to kettle and cook for 10 minutes.

5. Remove from heat. Just before serving, blend in yogurt. Add sea salt, if using, to taste. Top with parsley, if using.

CUCUMBER AVOCADO GAZPACHO

"Cool and creamy, the cucumber and avocado pair perfectly for a glorious summertime soup."

Servings: 4

Ingredients:

1 medium avocado, fully ripened

1 cucumber, peeled and seeds removed

1 clove garlic, minced

2 scallions

1 1/4 teaspoon sea salt

1 tbsp lime juice

1/2 tsp paprika

1 1/2 cups water (as needed)

1 sprig fresh basil (optional)

Directions:

1. Refrigerate all ingredients until very cold.

2. Put all ingredients into a blender and purée until smooth, adding water until desired consistency is reached.

3. Return the soup to the refrigerator and chill until ready to serve.

4. Garnish with a cucumber curl and fresh basil, if using.

Note: This recipe works best with a very powerful blender. You may want to coarsely chop your ingredients beforehand to get the right consistency.

GARLICKY SAUTÉED KALE

"Come and get your greens here! This recipe is easy and fast to make and loaded with good-for-you greens."

Servings: 4

Ingredients:

1 large bunch of kale

2 tbsp olive oil

5 cloves garlic, minced

Sea salt, to taste

Directions:

1. Tear kale into chunks and remove the stiffer stems.

2. Heat olive oil in a large skill over medium-high heat. Add garlic and stir for one minute.

3. Add kale and toss in skillet to coat with oil and garlic. Sprinkle with sea salt, if using. Cook for 1 to 2 minutes, or until kale is wilted but still crisp.

4. Remove from heat and serve.

PAD THAI SALAD

"This recipe takes the classic Pad Thai flavors and makes a delicious salad with lots of crunch and a nice ginger dressing."

Servings: 1

Ingredients:

1 tbsp coconut oil

1 egg

1 1/2 tbsp lime juice

1 clove garlic, minced

1/4 teaspoon ground ginger

2 tbsp almond butter

2 - 3 tbsp coconut or almond milk

1 tbsp. extra-virgin olive oil

Sea salt

1 cup cabbage, shredded

2 cups mixed greens

1/2 green bell pepper, sliced

1/2 cup broccoli sprouts

2 green onions, chopped

Directions:

1. In a small skillet, heat coconut oil over medium heat. Add egg and scramble while cooking for 3 to 4 minutes or until egg is done. Remove from heat and set aside.

2. In a small bowl, combine lime juice, garlic, ginger, almond butter, coconut milk and olive oil. Add sea salt to taste.

3. In a small bowl combine remaining ingredients and add cooled scrambled egg.

4. Pour dressing mixture over salad and serve.

Note: You can make more salad dressing and save the leftover dressing in a sealed container in your refrigerator for up to one week.

OVEN ROASTED ASPARAGUS

"Roasting asparagus with garlic and sea salt lends an aroma to the kitchen that will make you want to make this dish often."

Servings: 4

Ingredients:

1 bunch asparagus spears, ends trimmed

3 tablespoons olive oil

2 cloves garlic, minced

1 tbsp sea salt

1 tablespoon lemon juice (optional)

Directions:

Preheat oven to 425 degrees F (220 degrees C).

1. Line baking sheet with tin foil. Place the asparagus evenly on baking sheet. Drizzle with the olive oil. Using a tong, roll the asparagus evenly in the oil to coat. Lay spears so they do not overlap. Sprinkle with garlic and salt.

2. Bake in the preheated oven until just tender, 12 to 15 minutes depending on thickness. Sprinkle with lemon juice, if using, just before serving

ASPARAGUS BEEF ROLLS

"These creamy and flavorful rollups are great for dinner or served as an appetizer. This recipe does contain goat cheese so is better suited later on in your diet."

Servings: 2

Ingredients:

8 medium size asparagus spears

4 thin slices deli beef roast

4 oil-packed sun-dried tomatoes

1/2 cup goat cheese, divided

4 fresh basil leaves

2 tbsp olive oil

Directions:

1. Steam or boil the asparagus until just softened. Set aside.

2. Spread 2 tablespoons of goat cheese on each slice of beef. Add 1 sundried tomato, 1 basil leaf and 1 asparagus spear to each beef slice.

3. Roll up the beef slice with the ingredients inside. Stick a toothpick through the roll to hold it together.

4. Add olive oil to frying pan and preheat to medium-high. Add beef rollups to pan and cook for 3 to 4 minutes per side, or until nicely seared and before cheese starts to melt out of rollup. Serve.

CHIPOTLE LIME SALMON

"A wonderful zesty spicy salmon that is very satisfying and incredibly easy to make."

Servings: 2

Ingredients:

8 ounce salmon fillet

1 tbsp olive oil

Juice from 1 lime

1/2 tsp sea salt

1/2 tsp ground chipotle

Directions:

Preheat oven to 350 F (177 C)

1. Rinse salmon and pat dry. Place salmon on baking sheet.

2. Brush salmon with olive oil. Cut lime in half and squeeze juice onto fillet. Sprinkle with sea salt and chipotle.

3. Bake salmon for 15 to 20 minutes, or until salmon is still moist but flakes easily with a fork.

ROSEMARY GARLIC CHICKEN

"Crispy roasted chicken with the robust flavor of garlic and rosemary will delight your senses."

Servings: 2

Ingredients:

2 tbsp coconut oil

2 chicken leg quarters

6 garlic cloves

2 tsp sea salt

1 sprig fresh rosemary

Directions:

Preheat oven to 425 F.

1. Add coconut oil to glass baking dish and put in oven during preheating just until coconut oil is liquid.

2. Rinse chicken and pat dry. Place chicken in baking dish. Turn chicken over to coat with oil. Leave chicken skin side up in baking dish.

3. Place garlic cloves around chicken. Sprinkle chicken with sea salt and rosemary leaves.

4. Bake for 45 minutes or until chicken is crispy and internal temperature reaches 165 degrees.

ROASTED STUFFED BELL PEPPERS

"A delicious entrée stuffed with quinoa and a host of vegetables and spices. For a stunning, colorful presentation to delight your guests, choose red, green, yellow and orange bell peppers.

Note: This recipe includes carrots which should be avoided during your cleansing stage. Substitute kohlrabi for the carrots. Add the carrots back into this recipe when your candida is under control.

Servings: 2

Ingredients:

1 cup uncooked quinoa

2 tablespoon extra-virgin olive oil, divided

1 red onion, chopped

1/2 pound shiitake mushrooms, sliced

1 cup chopped carrots

1 cup chopped red bell pepper

6 bell peppers, tops removed, cored and seeded

1/2 cup chopped parsley

1/4 pound baby spinach

1 1/2 teaspoon ground cinnamon

3/4 teaspoon ground cumin

1/4 teaspoon fine sea salt

1. Cook quinoa according to package directions. Set aside to cool.

2. Heat oil in a large skillet over medium high heat. Add onion and cook, stirring occasionally until transparent. Add mushrooms and cook until softened. Add carrots and chopped peppers, cook until just softened. Add parsley and spinach. Let spinach wilt then stir in cinnamon, cumin and cooked quinoa and toss gently to combine. Add salt and cook 1 to 2 minutes more. Set aside to let filling cool until just warm.

   Preheat oven to 350°F. Lightly oil a 9x13-inch baking pan. Divide quinoa mixture evenly among remaining 6 bell peppers, gently packing it down and making sure to fully fill each pepper. Top each pepper with its reserved top, if desired, then arrange them upright in prepared pan. Cover tightly with foil.

   Bake peppers for 1 hour, or until peppers are tender and filling is hot. Check peppers after 30 minutes for doneness and moisture. When done to your liking, remove from oven and serve.

SAVORY LAMB CHOPS

"Tender, juicy lamb chops with garlic and Herbs de Provence combine for a wonderfully delicious and easy to make entree."

Servings: 2

Ingredients:

4 lamb chops

2 large garlic cloves, cut in half

2 tbsp olive oil

Sea salt to taste

1 tbsp Herbs de Provence

Directions:

Preheat oven to 350 F.

1. Add an oven-safe wire cooling rack to bottom of glass baking dish.

2. Cut a small slice into top of each lamb chop; do not cut through. Place lamb chops onto wire rack in baking dish. Put 1 half garlic clove into cut on top of each chop.

3. Baste each chop with olive oil. Sprinkle with sea salt and Herbs de Provence.

4. Bake for 25 minutes, or until lamb is done to your liking and the internal temperature reaches 145 degrees. Let rest 3 minutes before serving.

TREATS ON THE CANDIDA DIET

One of the ways I keep to the Candida diet is to have a few things that are treats but not way off the diet. Though fruit is sugar, it is also a much slower burning sugar than refined cane sugar, honey or maple sugar which makes it not as useful to the candida.

So when I crave a treat I do something with fruit. One favorite for me during the berry season is to simply pour cream over berries. Even better is to add to the berries and cream some coconut butter. Coconut butter (and cream for that matter) are both good fats to have for so many things in the body and I find I crave sugar less when I get enough fat. Which in turn helps me stay on the candida diet.

Following is a recipe for fruit compote. Keep in mind that to keep to the candida diet it is important to only eat treats like this once in a while and not daily. It is also best to add treats like this in only when you are in maintenance mode, not when you are in the initial stages of the candida diet cleanse.

FRUIT COMPOTE

Servings: 2

Ingredients:

Two apples or pears cut in ½" pieces

1 Tablespoon ghee or butter

1/3 cup apple juice (1/4 for pears)

1/2 teaspoon cinnamon

1/2 teaspoon nutmeg

Pinch of salt

Dollop of yogurt or cream (optional)

Note: More time is needed for apples to cook compared to pears which is why I put in less apple juice.

You can also add cherries, mango, blueberries or other non-citrus fruits you prefer.

Directions:

1. In sauce pan heat ghee. Add spices and simmer for 1 minute. Add fruit and sauté for 1 to 2 minutes. Add apple juice. Simmer until the fruit is soft but not mushy.

2. Top with yogurt or cream, if using.

It is helpful to have some probiotics and enzymes before having any food but especially a treat.

Alma Williams

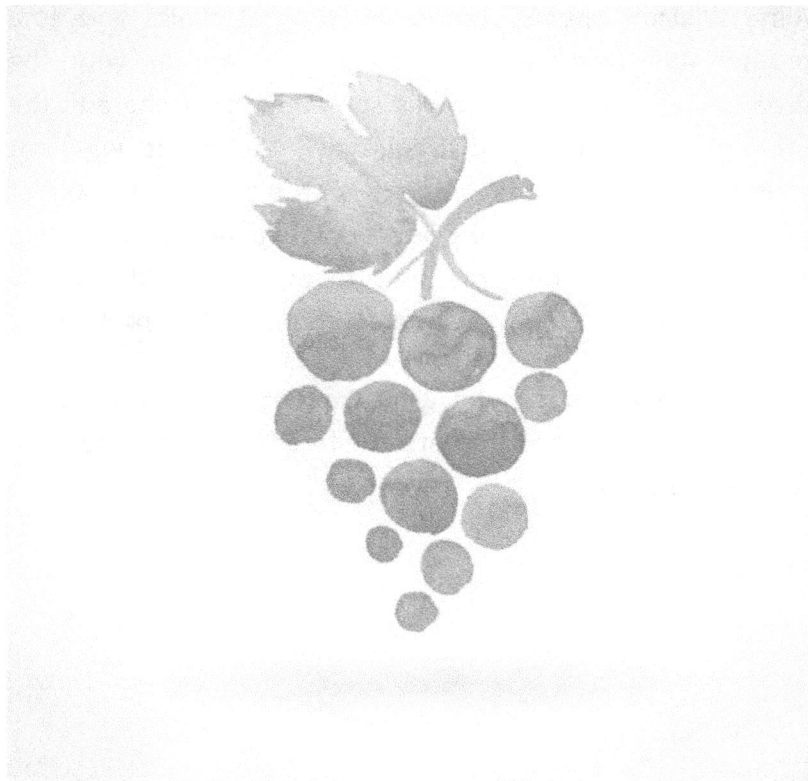

ABOUT THE AUTHOR

Alma Williams spent time volunteering at clinics and as a mother and daughter she was all too familiar with the dreaded yeast infection. It was something that she and the other females discussed frequently. Though it was not something that she was struggled with often, she knew that many women had recurring infections that seemingly had no cure. She started to do research to compile a guide to help women who were seeking viable solutions to their problem.

Her guide not only explains what Candida is but outlines the various methods and alternate treatments that can be used to cure the condition.

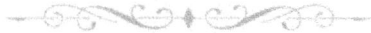